The ultimate weight loss hack :
Be healthy, new perspective on food , fitness and maintaining body shape

Latisha L. Johnson

INTRODUCTION

"The Ultimate Weight Loss Hack" reveals a game-changing technique to losing weight and achieving long-term fitness. In this ground-breaking book, the author takes a fresh look at the interwoven worlds of diet, fitness, and body shape maintenance. Beyond conventional dieting, the book reframes weight loss as a holistic journey, providing readers with a full arsenal for long-term success. It is jam-packed with practical insights that encourage people to ditch fad diets and live a healthy lifestyle. With a title that promises a weight reduction book that finally works, this fascinating read not only inspires but also provides readers with the tools they need to embark on a successful and long-term weight loss journey.

This isn't just another diet book; it's a trip into a world where health isn't a destination but a dynamic way of life. Prepare for a paradigm change as we reveal a fresh perspective on eating, fitness, and body shape maintenance. Instead of quick cures or restrictive plans, learn the art of building a complete well-being story.

We transcend the mundane in these pages, providing you with a refreshing approach that balances nutrition, exercise, and body positivity. It's not about being deprived; it's about being empowered. As you embark on this transforming journey, say goodbye to one-size-fits-all solutions and embrace personalised techniques that are tailored to your own experience. Prepare to rewrite the weight loss screenplay, where being healthy is not just a goal, but the ultimate and sustainable result. Let's begin this illuminating journey toward a healthier, more vibrant you.

Chapter 1

"A Fresh Start :The First Step To Creating A Healthier You"

The author's struggle for weight loss unfurled like a fascinating story in the battle of the bulge. The protagonist endured setbacks and cravings that read like plot twists while sweating it out in daily exercises and navigating a maze of mindful eating. Nonetheless, with unyielding resolve, each drop on the scale signified a thrilling chapter of triumph. Beyond a physical metamorphosis, the author discovered a powerful resilience narrative—a page-turner of self-discovery and the ultimate plot twist: rewriting the story of a healthier, happier life.

Benefits of adopting a healthy lifestyle

Adopting a healthy lifestyle yields a myriad of benefits. Improved physical well-being is evident through enhanced energy levels, weight management, and a strengthened immune system. Mental health receives a boost, reducing stress and promoting better mood and cognitive function. Long-term benefits include a lowered risk of chronic diseases such as heart conditions and diabetes. Additionally, adopting a healthy lifestyle fosters better sleep, increased productivity, and an overall sense of well-rounded fulfilment, creating a positive ripple effect across various facets of life.

Physical benefits

A healthy lifestyle has several physical advantages. Regular exercise helps with weight management, muscular and bone strength, and cardiovascular health. A well-balanced diet delivers critical nutrients that promote proper organ function and immune system vigour. Another important factor is adequate sleep, which benefits in physical recovery and overall well-being. Adopting healthy practices also lowers the chance of chronic diseases such as diabetes and hypertension, enhancing longevity. A physically active and nutritionally balanced lifestyle, in general, builds the groundwork for a resilient and vibrant body.

Mental and emotional benefits

Weight loss extends beyond the physical, encompassing significant mental and emotional benefits. As pounds drop, so does stress—exercise releases endorphins, acting as natural mood boosters. Enhanced body image and self-esteem accompany physical transformations, fostering a positive self-perception. The discipline required for weight loss cultivates mental resilience, positively impacting overall emotional well-being. Moreover, achieving weight loss goals often sparks a sense of accomplishment, reducing anxiety and depression. This holistic approach intertwines physical and mental health, creating a harmonious and empowered state of being.

Step in creating a healthier you in relationships to weight loss

Assessment and thing Setting: Estimate your current weight, health, and set realistic weight loss pretensions.

Nutritional Planning: Develop a balanced and sustainable diet, fastening on whole foods and portion control.

Physical exertion: Establish a regular exercise routine that includes both cardio and strength training.

Hydration: Prioritise acceptable water input, essential for overall health and supporting weight loss.

Sleep Optimization: Ensures sufficient and quality sleep to prop in recovery and regulate metabolism.

Stress operation: Utensil strategies to manage stress, as it can impact eating habits and weight.

Responsibility and Support: Engage with a support system, whether it's musketeers, family, or a weight loss group.

Monitoring: Progress Regularly track your weight, measures, and celebrate mileposts achieved.

aware Eating Practice aware eating, paying attention to hunger and fullness cues.

Rigidity: Be open to confirming your plan grounded on your body's response and life changes, fostering a sustainable approach to weight loss.

Chapter 2

"Nutrition: The Building Blocks Of A Healthy Diet"

A healthy diet necessitates a fundamental grasp of nutrition, eating behaviour, and the impact of your diet on your mental and physical well-being. Eating correctly can help you lose weight while also providing a number of core health benefits. The fundamentals of healthy eating may be learnt in a matter of minutes and will be extremely useful as you make appropriate diet options throughout medical weight loss.

Your eating habits influence your diet. These include the foods you choose, your response to hunger cues, when you eat, and how much you eat. While the term "diet" is commonly used to denote a short-term adjustment in eating habits that promotes weight reduction, a healthy diet is a long-term shift that encompasses fundamental changes in your eating patterns that promote continuous health and well-being.

What Exactly Is a Healthy Diet?

Your body relies on the meals you eat to provide nutrients, chemicals, and substances that serve as fuel for basic activities such as intellect, metabolism, and energy. Food nutrients are required for proper functioning and growth.

Nutrients are classified into six types:

Carbohydrates from protein
Vitamins and minerals
Water with Fat
All six of these nutrients are found in a well-balanced diet. When we don't obtain these nutrients, our bodies begin to shut down in what is known as a nutritional shortage. Dehydration

is an example of a dietary shortage caused by not drinking enough water.

Developing a Healthy Eating Habit
Creating a healthy diet necessitates numerous modifications in your eating habits. This includes changing the things you consume as well as some of your eating habits. Surround yourself with healthy foods as you work to develop a balanced diet. You can accomplish this by:

Eating a variety of whole foods. These are natural foods made from a single component. Fruits, vegetables, meats, nuts, and grains such as rice are all examples.
Making the switch to whole grains. Replace refined grains like sugar and white bread with whole grain brown rice and whole wheat bread to cut back on processed grains. Whole grains are high in fibre, which promotes metabolic health and digestion.
I'm drinking water. To stay hydrated, aim for 64 ounces of water every day. While other

beverages might keep you hydrated, they are generally high in calories and sugar. Juices and sodas with a lot of sugar should be avoided.

When developing a healthy diet, try to focus on the nutrients you are obtaining rather than the items you are avoiding. This might assist you in maintaining a good attitude toward creating a healthy diet.

Make every effort to prevent overeating. This can be accomplished by implementing healthy eating habits such as:

Maintaining reasonable portion sizes
Examining food labels
Avoiding thoughtless and emotional eating
reducing unnecessary calories

Following a healthy diet has numerous health benefits. A healthy diet lowers the risk of chronic diseases such as type 2 diabetes and heart disease. Good diet also aids in the stabilisation of cholesterol and blood sugar levels. A nutritious diet can naturally increase your energy, enhance your mood, and help you sleep better.

Avoiding processed or canned food .

Processed foods, often known as convenience or pre-prepared foods, are thought to contribute to the obesity pandemic and the increased prevalence of chronic diseases such as heart disease and diabetes.
Not all processed foods are unhealthy. Some foods must be processed to be safe, such as milk, which must be pasteurised to remove hazardous bacteria. A healthy diet can also include high-fibre morning cereals, wholemeal breads, and low-fat yoghurts.

Other foods require processing to be usable, such as pressing seeds to generate oil.

What makes certain processed foods unhealthy? Ingredients like salt, sugar, and fat are occasionally added to processed meals to improve their flavour and shelf life, or in some circumstances to contribute to the food's structure, like salt in bread or sugar in cakes.

People who buy processed foods may consume more than the recommended quantities of sugar, salt, and fat because they are unaware of how much has been added to the meal they are purchasing and eating.

These foods may also be higher in calories due to excessive levels of added sugar or fat.

You have no control over how important swab, sugar, and fat are in reused foods, but you do have control over what you buy. Examining food markers can help you choose between reused foods and keep track of the fat, swab, and sugar quantities. The nutrition information for utmost pre-packaged goods can be set up on the front, back, or side of the packaging. still, you will generally see a blend of red, amber, If the reused food you wish to buy has a colour- enciphered nutrition marker. still, look for further flora and ambers and lower reds when comparing analogous products, If you want to make a healthier choice. There are rules for determining if a food is high or low in fat, impregnated fat, swab, or sugar.

The guidelines for grown-ups are as follows: High total fat further than 17.5 g of fat per 100g Low 3g of fat per 100g or lower impregnated adipose acid further than 5g of impregnated fat per 100g is considered high. Low 1.5 g of impregnated fat per 100g or lower High sugar content further than 22.5 g total sugars per 100g Low 5g or lower of total sugars per 100g swab further than 1.5 g of swab per 100g(or0.6 g sodium) is considered high. Low 0.3 g or lower of swab per 100g(or0.1 g sodium). Still, strive to circumscribe your input of foods with further than 5g of impregnated fat per 100g, If you are trying to cut back on impregnated fat. Still, you should cut back because there's a correlation between red and reused meat and colon cancer, If you eat a lot of red or reused meat. We're encouraged not to consume further than 70g of sugar every day.

Food stuff to help you maintain weight

Eating nutrient-dense meals like lean protein and lentils can improve your overall health and help you lose weight.

While weight loss is not a panacea for health and is not for everyone, it may be something you want to aim toward in order to feel your best. Just make sure to consult with a doctor before making any significant changes.

If losing weight is your objective, these 16 foods may aid in your weight loss quest.
•Egg.
•Whole grain
•Chilli pepper
•Fruit
•Chia seeds
•Full fat
•leafy green
•Fish
•Cruciferous vegetables
•Chicken breast and some lean meats

•Potatoes and other root vegetables

•Beans and legumes

•Soup

•Cottage cheese

•Avocado

•Nut

Eating these nutritional reflections, together with temperance and regular exercise, should help pave the road to a healthy life

Specific Ingredients that are important for weight loss

Several nutrients have been linked as having the capability to prop in weight loss when included in a well- balanced diet. Then are a couple similar exemplifications

Green Tea Extract(EGCG Epigallocatechin Gallate)
It contains antioxidants and catechins, which may help to ameliorate metabolism and burn fat.

Caffeine

Acts as a goad, adding metabolic rate and physical performance while also helping to calorie burn.

Fibre

Reduces overall calorie consumption by promoting passions of wholeness. Fruits, vegetables, and whole grains are each high in fibre.

Protein

Supports muscle growth and form, increases passions of wholeness, and can help in the conservation of muscle mass during weight loss.

Chromium

Blood sugar situations may be regulated, potentially lowering jones and gluttony.

Calcium

According to some exploration, calcium-rich diets may prop in weight loss via affecting fat metabolism.

CLA(Conjugated Linoleic Acid)
CLA,which is set up in meat and dairy products, is allowed to have implicit benefits for weight loss and body composition.

Adipose Acids Omega- 3
Omega- 3 adipose acids, set up in adipose fish, chia seeds, and flaxseeds, may help reduce inflammation and promote general health during weight loss.

Glucomannan
Fibre that absorbs water and forms a gel- such as substance in the stomach, adding passions of wholeness and dwindling calorie input.

Capsaicin(deduced from chilli peppers)
Capsaicin, known for its metabolism- boosting rates, may contribute to enhanced calorie burn.

It's critical to flash back that, while these nutrients may give some backing, they aren't a phenomenal weight loss cure. A balanced and calorie- controlled diet, frequent physical exertion, and good life choices are essential for long- term weight loss. Before making significant changes to your diet or espousing supplements, always consult with a healthcare provider or a good dietitian.

Chapter 3

"The Power of hydration: How drinking Water Can Help You Lose Weight"

Staying hydrated is a crucial element in the realm of weight loss. Adequate water intake supports metabolism, aiding the body in burning calories more efficiently. Often, thirst can be mistaken for hunger, and staying hydrated helps distinguish between the two, preventing unnecessary snacking. Additionally, water can act as a natural appetite suppressant, promoting a feeling of fullness. Hydration also plays a vital role in energy levels, ensuring optimal performance during workouts. Ultimately, maintaining proper hydration is a cornerstone for overall well-being and successful weight loss.

The importance of staying hydrated and the health benefits of drinking enough water , including weight lose

Staying hydrated is essential for overall health, with specific weight-loss benefits:

Metabolic Boost: Hydration boosts metabolic functions, boosting the body's ability to burn calories efficiently.

Appetite Control: Water before meals can produce a sensation of fullness, reducing the likelihood of overeating and assisting with weight management.

Calorie-Free Hydration: Unlike sugary beverages, water has no calories, making it an excellent alternative for quenching thirst without increasing calorie intake.

Improved Exercise Performance: Hydration improves physical performance, allowing for more effective and sustained exercises, which is an important component of weight loss regimens.

Detoxification: Water aids in the removal of toxins from the body, assisting the liver and kidneys in their detoxification functions.

Fluid Balance: Maintaining fluid equilibrium in the body is critical for cellular function, nutrition transfer, and temperature regulation.

Increased Energy Levels: Dehydration can cause exhaustion and a decrease in energy levels. Staying hydrated ensures that you have enough energy for your regular activities and workouts.

Reduced Water Retention: Contrary to popular belief, good hydration can aid in water retention by indicating to the body that it is okay to release surplus fluids.

Water promotes digestion and reduces constipation, contributing to a healthy digestive tract, which is essential for proper nutrition absorption.

Skin Health: Hydration is essential for glowing skin, and well-hydrated skin is less prone to stretching, resulting in a better appearance after weight loss.

Explaining How much water to drink each day and how to make sure you're getting enough

In essence, drinking adequate water is a multidimensional technique that supports both general well-being and specific weight loss goals.

The appropriate amount of water to drink depends on factors such as age, weight, activity level, and climate. The "8x8 rule," which suggests eight 8-ounce glasses of water per day, totaling around 2 litres or half a gallon, is a generally suggested recommendation. Individual requirements, however, may vary.

To ensure you're receiving enough water, do the following:

Pay Attention to Your Body: Take note of thirst cues. Drink water if you're thirsty.

Consider Activity Levels: Physical activity requires more water. Drink more if you're working out.

Check Urine Colour: Pale yellow urine indicates adequate hydration, however dark yellow pee may indicate dehydration.

Climate: Increased water intake may be required to compensate for fluid loss through sweating in hot or humid conditions.

Hydrating Foods: Consume water-rich foods such as fruits and vegetables to help with overall hydration.

Carry a Water Bottle: Keep a reusable water bottle on you at all times for quick access.

Set timed Goals: for drinking water, such as before meals or at regular intervals throughout the day.

Use Apps or Reminders: Smartphone apps can track water consumption and provide reminders to stay hydrated.

Infuse with Flavor: To add flavour to ordinary water, infuse it with fruits, herbs, or a splash of citrus.

Increase Gradually: If you're not hitting your daily water targets, gradually increase your intake to allow your body to acclimate.

Staying hydrated is ultimately a personal journey. Adjust your water intake to fit your specific needs, taking into account the different elements that influence hydration.

Staying hydrated is a powerful ally in your weight loss journey. Adequate water intake supports metabolism, aids in appetite control, and enhances energy levels for effective workouts. Aim for about 8 glasses (64 ounces) a day, adjusting based on individual needs, activity levels, and climate. Pay attention to your body's thirst signals, monitor urine colour, and make hydration a consistent habit. Water's calorie-free simplicity makes it an ideal beverage choice, promoting fullness and aiding overall weight loss efforts.

Hydration takes centre stage as your loyal companion in the delicate dance of weight loss. Consider water to be the choreographer of metabolic equilibrium, appetite regulation, and energy-boosting performances. Imagine each drop as a transformational note in a symphony of health and vigour as you sip. Hydration becomes a rhythmic journey toward your weight loss goals rather than just a routine. Accept it as the secret ingredient that propels you onward with each refreshing reminder that each glass brings you one step closer to a healthier, happier you.

Chapter 4

"The Benefits of Exercise: How Moving Your Body Can Help You Lose Weight"

Benefits of regular exercise to weight lose

Regular exercise is a potent catalyst for weight loss, offering a spectrum of benefits:

Calorie Burning: Engaging in physical activity burns calories, creating a calorie deficit essential for weight loss.

Metabolic Boost: Exercise increases metabolism, promoting efficient calorie utilisation even at rest.

Muscle Development: Strength training builds muscle, which enhances overall metabolism and contributes to a leaner physique.

Appetite Regulation: Exercise helps regulate appetite hormones, reducing cravings and promoting mindful eating.

Fat Loss: Aerobic exercise, like jogging or cycling, is effective for burning stored fat, aiding in weight reduction.

Improved Insulin Sensitivity: Regular exercise enhances insulin sensitivity, crucial for managing blood sugar levels and preventing weight gain.

Enhanced Mood: Physical activity stimulates endorphin release, reducing stress and emotional eating tendencies.

Increased Energy Expenditure: Intense workouts elevate post-exercise oxygen consumption (EPOC), leading to continued calorie burning after exercise.

Better Sleep Quality: Regular exercise promotes deeper sleep, vital for overall well-being and weight management.

Long-Term Weight Maintenance: Sustained exercise habits contribute to maintaining weight loss achievements over time.

Incorporating a well-rounded fitness routine into your weight loss journey not only enhances physical health but also supports mental well-being, making it a fundamental component of a holistic approach to shedding pounds.

Exercise is more than just a workout; it is a weight loss ally. It burns calories, boosts metabolism, and shapes lean muscle. Aside from the physical benefits, it reduces cravings, reduces stress, and improves general well-being. Consider it a transforming journey, with each session adding to a healthier, happier you. It's not only about losing weight; it's about adopting a way of life in which movement becomes a celebration of your strength and vitality.

Exercise offers numerous other benefits than helping you lose weight, similar as increased moodTrusted Source, stronger bonesTrusted

Source, and a lower riskTrusted Source of numerous habitual conditions. Then are the top eight weight- loss exercises.

Waking: Tromping For numerous newcomers, walking can be a practical way to exercise without feeling overwhelmed or having to acquire an outfit. It's also a low- impact drill, which means it's less likely to strain your joints. Walking becks

roughly 7.6 calories per nanosecond for a 140- pound(65- kilogram) person, according to the American Council on Exercise. Walking becks about 9.7 calories per nanosecond for a 180- pound(81- kg) person. A 12- week investigationA study of 20 fat women revealed that walking for 50- 70 twinkles three times per week reduced body fat and midriff circumference by1.5 and 1.1 elevation(2.8 cm), independently. To begin, strive to walk for 30 twinkles three to four times a week. As you gain fitness, you can gradationally increase the length or frequency of your walks.

Running or Jogging: Although they appear to be the same, the main distinction is that a jogging speed is frequently between 4- 6 mph(6.4-9.7 km/ h), and a running pace is less than 6 mph(9.7 km/ h). According to the American Council on Exercise, a 140- pound(65- kg) person burns around 10.8 calories per nanosecond jogging and 13.2 calories per nanosecond handling. When jogging, a 180- pound(81- kg) person burns roughly 13.9 calories per nanosecond and 17 calories per nanosecond when running. Experimenters discovered that jogging and handling can help burn visceral fat, also known as belly fat. This kind of fat wraps around your internal organs and has been linked to a variety of habitual affections similar to heart complaints and diabetes. Begin with jogging for 20- 30 twinkles three to four times a week. Still, try running on softer shells similar to a lawn, If jogging or running outdoors hurts your joints. numerous routes include erected- in bumper, which may be more comfortable for your joints. MOREFind out how to lose weight using the WellosTM system.

Cycling: Cycling is a non-weight-bearing, low- impact drill that's gentle on your joints. According to the American Council on Exercise, a 140- pound(65- kg) person burns roughly 6.4 calories per nanosecond cycling at a speed of 10 long hauls per hour(MPH). Cycling at 10 MPH burns roughly 8.2 calories per nanosecond for a 180- pound(81- kg) person. People who cycle constantly have advanced overall fitness, increased insulin perceptivity, and a lower threat of heart complaint, cancer, and death than those who don't cycle constantly, according to studies. Cycling is generally an out-of-door exercise, but numerous gymnasiums and fitness installations have stationary bikes that allow you to cycle while remaining indoors.

Strength Training: Weight training can help you gain strength and muscle mass while also adding your resting metabolic rate(RMR), or the number of calories your body burns at rest. According to the American Council on Exercise, a 140- pound(65- kg) person burns roughly 7.6 calories every nanosecond of weight training. Weight training becks

roughly 9.8 calories per nanosecond for a 180- pound person. A six- month studyAccording to Trusted Source, conducting 11 twinkles of strength- grounded conditioning three times per week led in a7.4 rise in metabolic rate. This increase was similar to burning 125 calories per day in this study. Yet another studyAccording to Trusted Source, 24 weeks of weight training resulted in a 9% increase in men's metabolic rate, which equates to burning around 140 redundant calories each day. The increase in metabolic rate among women was roughly 4, or 50 redundant calories per day. Likewise, studies have shown that, as compared to aerobic exercise, your body continues to burn calories for numerous hours after a weight- training exertion.

Interval Exercise: Interval training, also known as high intensity interval training(HIIT), is a wide term for short bursts of ferocious exertion followed by rest intervals. A HIIT drill generally lasts 10- 30 twinkles and can burn a lot of calories. One exploration of 9 active males revealed that HIIT burnt 25- 30 further calories per nanosecond than other types of conditioning, similar as weight training, cycling, and routine jogging. That is, HIIT can help you burn further calories while doing lower exercise. multitudinous studies have indicated that HIIT is particularly effective for reducing abdominal fat, which has been linked to a variety of habitual conditions. To begin, select a kind of exercise, similar to running, jumping, or biking, as well as your drill and rest durations. For illustration, on a bike, pedal as hard as you can for 30 seconds, also sluggishly for 1- 2 twinkles. This pattern should be repeated for 10- 30 twinkles.

Swimming: According to the American Council on Exercise, swimming at a bottleneck or moderate pace becks

roughly 9 calories per nanosecond for a 140- pound(65- kg) person. Swimming at a bottleneck or moderate pace becks

about 11.6 calories per nanosecond for a 180- pound(81- kg) person. The quantum of calories you burn appears to be affected by how you swim. According to one study on competitive insensibility, the breaststroke burned the utmost calories, followed by the butterfly, backstroke, and freestyle. One 12- week exploration studySwimming for 60 twinkles three times per week for 24 middle-aged women dramatically reduced body fat, better inflexibility, and reduced colourful heart complaint threat factors, including high total cholesterol and blood triglycerides, according to a study published in Trusted Source. Swimming is low- impact, which means it's gentler on your joints. This makes it an excellent choice for anyone suffering from injuries or common discomfort.

Yoga: While yoga isn't generally allowed As a weight loss drill, it does burn a significant quantity of calories and provides multitudinous redundant health advantages that can prop in weight loss. A 12- week investigationA study of 60 fat women revealed that those who shared in two 90- nanosecond yoga sessions per week endured advanced midriff circumference reductions than those in the control group — by and normal of 1.5 elevation(3.8 cm).

The yoga group also saw earnings in their internal and physical well- being. Yoga, in fact, has been proved in studies to educate awareness and reduce stress situations. Yoga classes are available at most gymnasiums , but you can exercise yoga anywhere. This includes working from home, as there are multitudinous guided assignments available online.

Pilates:. An individual importing roughly 140 pounds(64 kg) would burn 108 calories in a 30- nanosecond freshman's Pilates session or 168 calories in a 30- nanosecond intermediate class, according to a study patronised by the American Council on Exercise. Although Pilates doesn't burn as many calories as cardio exercises like running, it's further fun for numerous individuals, making it easier to keep to over time. An eight- week studyIn a study of 37 middle-aged women, Trusted Source discovered that completing Pilates movements for 90 twinkles three times per week significantly reduced midriff, stomach, and hipsterism circumference when compared to a control group that conducted no exercise during the same time period. Pilates may also help you lose weight.Dependable source reduce back discomfort and enhanceStrength, balance, inflexibility, abidance, and total fitness from a reliable source. Pilates can be done at home or in one of the numerous gymnasiums that give Pilates assignments. Combine Pilates with a healthy diet and other forms of exercise, similar as weight training or cardio, to accelerate weight loss indeed further.

Leveraging bodyweight exercises is a strategic approach to weight loss. These exercises, such as squats, push-ups, and lunges, not only burn calories but also promote lean muscle development, fostering a more sculpted physique. Their versatility allows for customization, adapting to different fitness levels and ensuring consistent engagement. The full-body nature of many bodyweight exercises intensifies calorie burn and engages multiple muscle groups simultaneously, contributing to efficient fat loss. Incorporating these exercises into a routine enhances metabolism, creating a sustained calorie-burning effect. The convenience of bodyweight workouts, requiring minimal equipment, facilitates regularity, a vital component of successful weight loss. Embrace this accessible and adaptable fitness approach to not only shed pounds but to build a foundation for lasting health and wellness.

The Significance Of Setting Goals And Tracking Progress In Relation To Weight Loss.

Setting goals and tracking progress are important when it comes to losing weight through exercise:

1. Workouts with Specific Goals:

Why It's Important: Exercise goals that are clearly stated align with your weight loss aims, whether it's burning calories, developing muscle, or improving endurance.
How to Apply It: To keep workouts purposeful and effective, set specific training goals such as completing a certain number of reps, increasing running distance, or attempting new exercises.

2. Metrics of Performance:

Why It's Important: Goals provide milestones for success, transforming workouts into measurable gains.
How to Apply It: Keep track of your workout metrics, such as reps, weights, time, and distance. Assess and set new goals on a regular

basis to guarantee a progressive and demanding fitness routine.

3. Activity-Based Accountability:

Why it Matters: Setting exercise goals creates a sense of accountability, promoting continuous physical activity participation.
How to Apply It: Set weekly or monthly workout objectives and keep track of your progress. To increase accountability, share your goals with a workout buddy or use fitness apps.

4. Adaptation for Best Results:

Why it Matters: Regular evaluation helps you to tweak your workout regimen to maximise its influence on weight loss.
How to Apply It: If an activity isn't producing results, adjust the intensity, length, or attempt a different program. Adapting ensures that efficacy is maintained.

5. Physical Development and Motivation:

Why It's Important: Improving your exercise performance maintains the link between physical activity and weight loss.

How to Apply It: Use workout records, before-and-after images, or fitness apps to track your improvement. Celebrate accomplishments to keep motivation high.

6. Consistency in Exercise Habits:

Why It's Important: Setting and recording exercise goals creates a routine, which promotes consistency in weight loss efforts.

How to Apply It: Schedule regular workout sessions, keep track of your progress, and create a routine that will help you lose weight.

7. Movement for Mental Well-Being:

Why it Matters: Exercise progress boosts confidence, reduces stress, and adds to a positive outlook.

How to Apply It: Recognize and value how exercise improves your mental health, confirming the link between physical activity and overall weight loss success.

By combining exercise with weight loss goals, you develop a synergistic strategy in which each session becomes a meaningful step toward your ideal weight. Goal setting, tracking progress, and frequent exercise not only improves physical fitness but also propels you toward long-term and holistic weight loss.

How To Track Exercise Progress With A Journal Or Fitness App

Keeping a Journal

Set specific objects:

•Define your fitness objects easily. Having defined objects, whether for weight loss, muscle structure, or lesser abidance, will direct your shadowing.

Make a Workout Journal

•Keep track of the exercises, sets, reiterations, and weights used during each drill. Take note of the time and intensity of your cardio sessions.

Weights and measure

•Track physical changes by measuring crucial regions(midriff, hips,etc.) and noting your weight on a regular basis. Do this on a regular basis, similar to daily or biweekly.

Keeping a Food Journal

•Keep a food journal to track your eating habits. Keep track of what you eat, how important you eat, and any changes in your eating habits.

What You suppose

•Keep track of how you feel after each drill. Keep track of your energy situations, mood, and any changes in your overall well- being.

Prints of Progress

•Include images of progress at regular intervals. These visual signals serve as a physical representation of your experience.

Observe mileposts

•Fete accomplishments and mileposts. This could be reaching a specific weight, completing a delicate exertion, or setting a particular stylish

Consider and Acclimate

•Review your journal on a regular basis. Consider what's working and what needs to be better. Acclimate your pretensions and ways as demanded.

Making Use of a Fitness App

Elect an Applicable App

•Choose a fitness app that corresponds to your objects. numerous apps feed to different fitness situations and pretensions.

Produce Your Profile

•Enter your particular information, similar to age, weight, and fitness position. You may also establish particular fitness objects with some operations.

Drill Log Enter.

•Drill details similar to exercises, sets, reps, and weights. Some apps also include pre-programmed exercises.

Keep track of your nutrition

•Log your diurnal food consumption using the app's capabilities. numerous apps include vast food and nutritive database databases.

Track Progress Graphs

•Use the progress monitoring options, which constantly include graphs that show changes in weight, measures, or drill performance over time.

Wearable Device Sync

•Sync your fitness shamus or smartwatch with the app. This ensures that way, heart rate, and other essential parameters are directly tracked.

Receive Reminder and Challenges

•Monuments and challenges will be transferred to you numerous apps give monuments for exercises, water consumption, and mess medication. Some offer challenges to keep you motivated.

Join the Community

•Join the app's community or connect with musketeers who are also using the app. Participating accomplishments and progress might help to make provocation.

A journal and a fitness app are both useful for tracking progress. Choose the strategy that stylish suits your interests and life, and use it as a tool to track and celebrate your fitness trip on a regular basis.

Chapter 5

"Mind over matter :The Psychology of Weight Loss"

" Mind over matter in weight loss psychology emphasises the important part of internal processes in achieving and maintaining a healthy weight." It emphasises the significance of provocation, thing planning, and aware eating practices. Individuals can overcome emotional eating, produce sustainable habits, and negotiate problems by cultivating a happy mindset. The approach recognizes that losing weight is further than just a physical exercise; it also necessitates a thorough mindfulness of one's own conduct, feelings, and internal patterns. employing the mind's eventuality allows for holistic and long-term metamorphosis, with a focus on tone-efficacy and the cerebral.

The psychology of weight reduction involves a complicated interaction of behaviours, emotions, and cognitive processes. Understanding these psychological components is essential for designing long-term and effective weight-management techniques. The following are crucial elements:

Motivation
•*Intrinsic vs. Extrinsic Motivation:* Internal motivations, such as improved health or more energy, tend to be more sustainable than external motives, such as societal standards.

Setting goals:
•*Smart Goal:* Specific, Measurable, Achievable, Relevant, and Time-bound goals help build a clear roadmap for achievement.

Eating With Intention:
•*Mindfulness:* Practising mindfulness during meals promotes a healthier relationship with food, promoting better choices and preventing overeating.

Emotional Eating

•Recognizing Triggers: Identifying emotional triggers for overeating and developing alternate coping methods is critical for ending the cycle.

Self-Efficacy:
•Belief in Ability: Developing confidence in your ability to make healthy choices and conquer problems is critical for long-term success.

Positive Reinforcement:
•Celebrating Progress: Recognizing and celebrating little accomplishments enhances motivation and reinforces the link between effort and success.

Self-Compassion:
•Self-Compassion: Practising self-compassion minimises negative self-talk and creates a positive outlook, which is essential during setbacks.

Behavioural Trends:

•*Identifying Habits:* Recognizing and changing unhealthy habits gradually and sustainably is more successful than sudden adjustments.

Social Assistance:
•*Impact on the Community:* Connecting with a supportive community or requesting help from friends and family provides encouragement and accountability.

Stress Reduction:
•*Healthy Coping Strategies:* Developing non-food-related stress coping skills lowers the chance of emotional eating.

Cognitive Reorganisation:
•*Changing Thought Patterns:* Changing negative thought patterns regarding food and body image promotes a healthier mentality.

Integrating Your Lifestyle:
•*Sustainability:* Choosing adjustments that may be incorporated into daily life over time

increases the likelihood of weight reduction maintenance.

Remember that weight loss psychology is highly individual. Tailoring tactics to your own psychological profile, getting professional help when necessary, and approaching the process with patience and self-compassion all contribute to a more effective and long-term weight reduction experience.

How to Overcome Emotional Eating and How To Stay Motivated and Committed to Your Goal

Promoting emotional eating is pivotal for long-term weight loss success. relating triggers, promoting needed managing styles, and encouraging conservative eating actions all help to break the cycle of using food as a bolsterer for emotional discomfort. Staying motivated and devoted also includes setting realistic pretensions, relating natural provocations, and satisfying progress. Creating a probative terrain, holding oneself responsible, and incorporating variety into your habit all help to sustain provocation. individuals can develop a balanced and long- term weight loss approach by addressing both emotional aspects and commitment strategies.

How Our Minds Impact Our Eating Habit

Eating Emotionally: Calorie intake and weight are affected by emotional eating, which occurs when one gives in to one's emotions and eats more than one needs. For successful weight loss, it is essential to recognize and manage emotional eating.

Routines and habits: Eating poorly is a major contributor to consuming too many calories. Making deliberate decisions breaks habitual routines and encourages a change to better food choices and quantity management.

Mental Factors: Eating disorders can develop from persistently negative ideas about food or one's physique. In order to lose weight and keep it off, it's important to work on these mental components.

External Factors: Cultural and societal standards have the potential to impact dietary preferences and intake levels. Making educated decisions that support weight loss objectives is made easier with increased awareness.

Craving: To keep the caloric deficit required for weight loss, it is crucial to manage cravings, especially for meals that are high in calories. To overcome these cravings, practise mindful eating.

Decision-Making: Impulse control and effective decision-making impact dietary choices. Making careful, health-conscious decisions aids weight loss efforts.

Mind-Body Connection: Tuning into hunger and fullness cues aids in portion control and prevents overeating, key components of a successful weight loss journey.

Motivation and Goal Alignment: Intrinsic reasons, such as improved health, drive continuous efforts in weight loss. Aligning eating habits with weight loss objectives boosts commitment and success.

The interplay between our brains and eating habits is a fundamental component of the weight loss journey. Building awareness, making thoughtful decisions, and treating psychological problems contribute to a sustainable and holistic strategy to dropping pounds.

Weight reduction is strongly tied to the science of how our minds influence our eating habits and how emotions influence food choices. Here's how it's done:

Emotional Eating and Caloric Intake

Emotional moods can lead to overeating, which contributes to a calorie surplus. Emotional eating must be managed in order to sustain the essential calorie deficit for weight loss.
System of Food Reward:

System of Food Reward

Certain foods, particularly those high in sugar and fat, activate the reward system in the brain, resulting in cravings. Considering the neural aspects of reward can help you make more conscious dietary choices.

Hormonal Control and Hunger Signals

Emotional moods can disturb hormones that influence appetite and fullness, affecting portion management. Controlling these hormonal responses is critical for successful weight loss.

Overeating Caused by Stress

Cortisol release caused by stress can result in desires for comfort foods. Stress management and emotional response strategies are critical for avoiding stress-related overeating.

Making Decisions and Making Healthy Choices

Emotional stress can affect decision-making and contribute to the consumption of harmful meals. Weight loss objectives can be aided by cultivating awareness and skills for making health-conscious decisions.

Habit Conformation and exertion

Emotional moods can impact the development of dangerous eating actions. Addressing conditioned emotional responses aids in breaking weight loss tendencies. Intuitive

Eating and awareness

Awareness and intuitive eating are two practices that promote emotional and physiological mindfulness. This increased mindfulness allows for further deliberate and health-conscious eating selections.

Environmental and social factors

Emotional eating practices are constantly shaped by external forces and societal morals. Creating a terrain that encourages healthy choices aids in weight loss success.

Behavioural variations and Neuroplasticity

Purposeful adaptations in study and that make use of the brain's neuroplasticity help people establish healthier eating habits that lead to weight loss.

Overall Health and Weight Control

Addressing emotional and internal factors promotes a good outlook, adaptability, and a long- term approach to weight loss.

Understanding the scientific foundations of how our studies impact eating habits and feelings impact food choices is critical for developing effective, comprehensive weight loss and long- term well- being results.

Chapter 6

"The Art of Maintenance – Nurturing Your New Self Beyond the Finish Line"

When you reach the crossroads of achievement, having overcome the hurdles of weight reduction, the journey takes a powerful turn—you enter the domain of maintenance. This chapter is your guide to not just retaining your victories, but also prospering in the continuous story of your well-being. Join us as we delve into the complex artistry of maintenance, learning how to nurture the bright, transformed version of yourself and building the road for a future of lasting health and balance.

Habits of Longevity in Nutrition:

Transitioning from the thrilling pursuit of weight loss to the more delicate arena of weight maintenance necessitates a new perspective on diet. This part shows the way toward long-term eating habits that not only fortify your hard-won accomplishments but also serve as the foundation of a nourishing, long-lasting lifestyle.

Balanced Eating concepts: The adventure continues with a deep dive into the concepts of balanced eating. We investigate the profound influence of diversified, nutrient-dense foods on your overall health, rather than the pursuit of a number on the scale. It's about embracing a palette of colours and sensations that not only satisfy your taste senses but also nourish your body, allowing you to maintain your vigour.

Meal Planning for Maintenance: Meal planning takes centre stage in the arena of maintenance. But don't worry; this isn't about rigid patterns or monotony; rather, it's a celebration of gastronomic diversity personalised to your tastes. Discover how to create meal plans that seamlessly integrate into your lifestyle, ensuring a seamless marriage of health and fun. We go into the art of preparing meals that become a source of delight, thereby promoting your overall well-being.

Join us on this journey of sustainable nutrition, where the journey is about savouring each mouthful as you continue to nurture the masterpiece that is your transformed self.

Lifetime Fitness Routines:

As the path of maintenance continues, our focus shifts to fitness—a critical component in shaping a future of sustainable health and vitality. This section serves as your compass, guiding you through the ever-changing terrain of fitness regimens that not only preserve but also improve your physical health.

Workout Adaptation: Say goodbye to the rigidity of organised weight loss programs. The maintenance phase necessitates a fluid approach—an investigation of workouts customised to your changing objectives. Discover the joy of movement as we explore ways that adapt to your lifestyle and ensure consistency and effectiveness in every session.

Including Variety: The days of monotony are over. Maintenance encourages you to incorporate variety into your training activities. We reveal the several ways to make your workouts interesting, from yoga to strength training, cardio bursts to outdoor experiences. Accept variety as a source of inspiration and physical wellbeing, not just a means to an end.

Join us on this fitness journey where the desire of health meets the pleasure of exercise. It's time to develop a sustainable and pleasurable habit that will go beyond the finish line, ensuring that fitness is a lifelong partner in your wellness journey.

Navigating Difficulties:

Challenges are unavoidable in the ongoing story of maintenance, but they are also stepping stones to resilience and long-term success. This part will teach you how to overcome obstacles and emerge stronger on the other side.

Resolving Obstacles: No trip is without its challenges, and upkeep is no exception. Learn how to deal with setbacks with grace and resilience. Learn how to pivot and recommit to your well-being goals in the face of a brief slip in healthy behaviours or unexpected life circumstances.

Building Resilience: Resilience is the foundation of effective maintenance. Explore the skill of bouncing back stronger, building a mindset that sees problems as opportunities for growth rather than obstacles. Learn to accept setbacks as a necessary part of the path, confirming your dedication to long-term well-being.

Join us in this investigation of resilience, where setbacks become catalysts for continuing growth and every setback serves as an opportunity to progress further on your maintenance path.

Milestones to Remember:

Take time to celebrate your achievements that go beyond the scale as you continue your journey of maintenance. This section recognizes the tremendous influence of your dedication on numerous elements of your life and celebrates successes that go beyond numerical measurements.

Non-Scale Victories: Move away from the scale and into a domain where victories are more than just numbers. Experience the thrill of more energy, better sleep, improved attitude, and a fresh confidence that emanates from inside. Recognize and celebrate these non-scale successes as significant indicators of your general well-being.

Self-Reflection: Take a moment to reflect on your transformational path. This part invites you to reflect, recognizing your personal progress, learning, and good improvements. Self-reflection is a strong tool for reaffirming your commitment to long-term well-being and appreciating your journey.

Celebrate the several victories that lead to a comprehensive sense of accomplishment. It's time to acknowledge the fundamental changes in your life, understanding that true achievement in maintenance goes well beyond the statistics, cultivating a lasting sense of fulfilment and pride in your well-being journey.

Integrating Your Lifestyle:

Maintenance is not a distinct phase; it is the seamless incorporation of good practices into the fabric of your daily life. This section looks at how to make well-being a natural part of your daily routine, so that your dedication to health becomes second nature.

Daily Sustainability: Learn the skill of making health-conscious choices a natural part of your daily routine. From morning rituals to bedtime routines, we look at ways to easily include diet, exercise, and self-care into your daily routine. Discover the delight of sustainability as your health and well-being become woven into the fabric of your being.

Balancing Act: Explore the delicate balance between work, relationships, and personal well-being in the Balancing Act. This section goes into ways for keeping balance in a world that frequently demands a lot. Learn how to prioritise self-care without sacrificing other elements of your life, ensuring that your journey of maintenance contributes to your overall satisfaction rather than detracts from it.

Begin your journey into lifestyle integration, where health is not a chore but an essential part of who you are. It's time to develop a balanced and meaningful life in which every decision contributes to your long-term happiness.

It is critical to maintain your body after a successful weight loss journey to avoid reverting to prior shapes. The importance is in consolidating your hard-earned accomplishments and cultivating long-term habits. Maintenance isn't a one-time event; it's a continuous commitment to the lifestyle adjustments that fueled your transformation. You develop a buffer against the return of old behaviours by persistently practising healthy eating, remaining physically active, and nurturing your general well-being. It's about accepting a new normal—one that stresses health and recognizes the cyclical nature of happiness. Without this commitment, the chance of regaining weight looms. As a result, the value of maintenance extends far beyond aesthetics; it is a shield against the traps of complacency, ensuring that the journey toward long-term health becomes a lifelong adventure rather than a fleeting victory.

CONCLUSION

In the big finale of "The Ultimate Weight Loss Hack: Be Healthy," we conclude not only a book, but a transforming journey into a more vibrant, healthier you. As we say goodbye to these pages, keep in mind that this is just the beginning. The path to excellent health goes beyond these words, resonating in the decisions you make and the habits you form.

Accept your newfound perspective on diet, fitness, and body form. It is not about perfection, but rather about growth. Each chapter served as a stepping stone to a more holistic understanding of well-being. You're not simply armed with information; you're also empowered to personalise your health path.

So, as you go, let this book be a companion, a reference, and a reminder that staying healthy is an ongoing process. Celebrate every accomplishment, eat every balanced meal, and enjoy every active moment. The ultimate weight reduction trick has been revealed: living a life where health is not a destination but an ever-changing, joyful journey toward your ideal self. Here's to your next adventure—may it be as gratifying and exciting as the new viewpoint you've adopted.